1990

SELF-ESTEEM BUILDING

A Guide for Parents and Professionals Working with Persons with Developmental Disabilities

Roger A. Frank
Rehabilitation Guidance Counselor
Portland Community College
and
Private Practice Counselor
Portland, Oregon

Jean P. Edwards
Professor, Special Education
Portland State University
Portland, Oregon

i

ACKNOWLEDGEMENTS

Our thanks to Roger "Opie" Parker for all his help with this book. His practical help and encouragement was very much appreciated. We hope the next book will be his own!

Cover photo: John Stewart. Judy Cunio gives her first formal speech before an audience of more than 1000 PEOPLE FIRST members.

Laser Typesetting: Carolyn Bradley
Editing and Proofing: Molly Emmons

Library of Congress Card Catalog Number: 88-83300
International Standard Book Number: 0-944480-04-17
Printed in the United States of America

DEDICATION

First, we would like to dedicate this book to the
memory of our grandmother

Beatrice Putnam

who inspired us with her love, hope and courage,
as well as her own self-esteem.

And to our friends

Pat and Louise Highhouse

Their personal and professional competencies have
been a source of great strength to our lives.

Louise radiates inner beauty;
Pat self-responsibility and goal setting.

Both are excellent role models as
parents
professionals
and friends.

TABLE OF CONTENTS

Introduction

Part I The Need for Self-Esteem

Part II   Strategies for Promoting Self-Confidence

Part III   Strategies for Enhancing Self-Respect

Appendices

INTRODUCTION

Most parents and professionals would do anything they could to ensure that a child with developmental disabilities could grow up happy, healthy and successful at a job and at independent living.

Most want for that child a happy home life, close friends and financial security.

Though we invest our time, energy and financial resources in doing many things to enhance the quality of life for persons with developmental disabilities, we do far too little to improve self-esteem, the most crucial key to the psychological well-being of all persons.

We hope that this book will be a source of great encouragement and practical help to parents and professionals ready to acknowledge that self-esteem is the most significant key to our behavior, our successes, and our ability to face disability.

It is never too late to boost a person's self-esteem!

Part I

The Need for Self-Esteem

Chapter I

WHAT IS SELF-ESTEEM?

Positive self-esteem is the capacity to view oneself with a fundamental sense of value and competence. It is the inner belief that we can meet the challenges of our existence. Healthy self-esteem is an essential human need and crucial to our psychological well-being. Humanistic psychologist Abraham Maslow (1954, p. 45) explained the importance of self-esteem in this way:

> "Satisfaction of the self-esteem need leads to feelings of self-confidence, worth, strength, capability, and adequacy, of being useful and necessary in the world. But thwarting of these needs produces feelings of inferiority, of weakness and of helplessness."

Without self-esteem our psychological survival is threatened and the very foundations of our self-structure weaken and erode. The importance of thinking of ourselves in healthy, positive ways cannot be underestimated. Self-esteem profoundly influences our thinking processes, interpersonal relationships, career choices, and the sense of control we have over our lives.

Much has been written in the past few years regarding how our thinking processes affect our feelings and self-esteem. It is generally accepted that our beliefs or outlook regarding a certain event will greatly influence our feelings or emotions about that event. For example, someone calls us on the phone and breaks a date. Our immediate reaction will probably depend on how important that person is to us and what the circumstances were surrounding cancellation of the date. But our reaction may also be dependent on our level of self-esteem. If we have low self-esteem our beliefs or outlook may cause us to say things like, "I don't have any friends," "I'm such a loser," "The world is no damn good." Our emotions following that kind of negative self-talk will probably include feelings of rejection, sadness, loneliness and low self-esteem. If we have high self-esteem we will most likely interpret the event differently and our self-talk may include "This won't be a problem, I'll simply call someone else," or "I can handle this, I'll read a book or watch television tonight." Our emotional reaction will be more calm and controlled and may only include mild sadness or disappointment. The distinction involves how our level of self-esteem affects our outlook or beliefs. People with low self-esteem have more of a tendency to overreact, overgeneralize, and make "mountains out of molehills." They may also be excessively self-critical and self-blaming due to their feelings of inadequacy and unworthiness. Individuals with high self-esteem will generally react in a more reasonable, rational way. Their feelings of self-worth and value help them to better handle disappointments or setbacks.

Self-esteem also plays a major role in the success of our interpersonal relationships. The idea that "If you don't love yourself you can't love someone else" has become something of a cliche these days. It is true, but let's take it a step further. If we don't love ourselves, if we have truly low self-esteem, then it would be very difficult to believe that someone else could love us. We wouldn't experience their commitment or devotion as convincing because we feel basically unlovable. Deep down, our self-talk may include statements like, "Why does this person love me?" "I have nothing to offer anyone." "What do they really want?" Questioning the other person's motives, as well as our own self-worth, can eventually lead to the downfall of relationships. People with low self-esteem are often excessively jealous, possessive, manipulative, and controlling. They also require constant reassurances that they are okay, especially from those closest to them. Individuals with healthy, positive self-esteem have an inner joy and sensitivity that improves the quality of relationships. Instead of being suspicious and domineering they are generally more trusting and flexible. As a result the relationship progresses to a deeper level wherein intimacy and mutual respect are enhanced.

The biggest roadblock to career success and achievement is not believing in ourselves and our abilities. We choose careers based on an assessment, usually subjective, of our strengths, skills, and talents. If our self-esteem is low then the career we choose will usually reflect an underestimation of our abilities. The resulting job will probably fail to challenge or stimulate and the cycle of low self-esteem will continue. Persons with high self-esteem generally choose careers which involve greater complexity and higher goals. Because they feel a fundamental sense of competency and worth, they trust in their ability to handle difficult challenges. On the job they put out extra effort and continually search for the most innovative and effective ways to carry out the tasks they've been given. To them the job is an opportunity to succeed and grow. On the job the person with low self-esteem adheres rigidly to the policies and procedures they were initially taught. They rarely seek out new ways to perform the job and instead choose to stick with what's safe and familiar. This tendency to play it safe and avoid risks and demanding goals is an important distinction between those individuals with high and low self-esteem.

A lack of self-esteem, as Maslow noted, can lead to feelings of inadequacy and helplessness. Persons with low self-esteem often do feel a sense of helplessness or loss of control over their environment. Because they have no sense of personal competency or efficacy, they avoid making choices or decisions. When faced with problems or setbacks they typically complain that they were "the victim of circumstances" or that it was "the other guy's fault."

By avoiding responsibility for their actions (or inactions) such individuals feel helpless and ineffective and, in so doing, continually reinforce a negative self-evaluation. On the other hand, persons with high self-esteem feel they can significantly influence their environment. Trusting in their inner resources allows them to take charge of their lives. They recognize that we as human beings have free will and that we are responsible for our choices and actions. When the awareness of self-responsibility is understood and exercised, then one feels much more control and self-esteem is greatly enhanced.

Chapter II

WHY SELF ESTEEM IS ESSENTIAL FOR INDIVIDUALS WITH DEVELOPMENTAL DISABILITIES

Healthy, positive self-esteem is important for everyone but it is essential for people with disabilities. Clearly, life is difficult. But life is especially hard if one has a developmental or physical disability. One of this book's authors is in a wheelchair due to a spinal injury fourteen years ago. I speak from experience in saying there are many frustrations, inconveniences, and barriers for persons with disabilities. Our society has a long way to go in terms of attitudes and accessibility. Overcoming a disability of any kind takes a great deal of patience, persistence, and guts. Positive self-esteem provides an invaluable edge. It helps us to "roll with the punches" and bounce back from failure or setbacks. Self-esteem is the inner conviction that we can rise above adversity. Without a doubt, the single most significant factor in the adjustment to my own disability has been my feelings of personal worth and adequacy.

For the adolescent or young adult with a developmental disability, healthy self-esteem can lead to increased independence, spontaneity, happiness and productivity. It is an inner emotional wealth that they can channel into their relationships, work, and goals and dreams for the future. Self-esteem also adds to personal empowerment, greatly increasing the effectiveness of assertiveness training and other techniques for avoiding exploitation. Without self-esteem the stigmatizing effects of a developmental disability are amplified and we are more subject to feelings of shame, self-doubt, uncertainty and confusion. There are many variables which contribute to low self-esteem in individuals with developmental disabilities. Some can be traced to childhood and parenting practices while others reflect an inability of our communities to develop adequate individual and family counseling services. Additional factors stem from cultural attitudes and others can be linked to the labels and categories we assign to the disability itself. These variables which diminish self-esteem in persons with developmental disabilities include overprotection and isolation, myths and discrimination, labeling and devaluation, and a lack of adequate mental health counseling and services.

Overprotection and Isolation

Overprotection of the child with a developmental disability due to low expectations will hinder growth and maturity. If the child is not encouraged to take risks and test his or her abilities, overdependence and helplessness will result. On the other hand, overly high expectations resulting in frustration and failure may cause the development of a "quitter" self-image. In this circumstance the child does not learn persistence and determination, two very important qualities which are essential for healthy self-esteem. Special attention should be given in order to determine what limitations there are, and what strengths and abilities exist. Repeated trials and continuous reassessments will be needed to find out what is achievable, then goals can be set and realistic expectations can be established.

Many parents may be told by less understanding physicians to institutionalize their disabled child at birth or that "he may not walk or talk until three or four or never." These comments are shattering and often prompt protective behaviors and limit parental expectations early.

Isolation of the child or adolescent with a developmental disability will also lead to poor self-esteem. Parents and nondisabled siblings may isolate children with disabilities from friends and neighbors due to feelings of shame and embarrassment. Isolation may also occur if there is a shortage of community resources for persons with developmental disabilites. Such resources would include opportunities for leisure, recreation, and social interaction. The child's self-esteem will most certainly suffer if he feels no value as a family member, has little or no social interaction, and has no real opportunity to explore the outside world.

Myths and Discrimination

Myths generate barriers to progress. They create roadblocks to societal acceptance of persons with developmental disabilities. One such common myth states that "developmentally disabled people have short attention spans and therefore cannot learn anything." Of course we know that people learn in diferent ways. Through proper training and careful task analysis, individuals with developmental disabilities can do many things. They can be taught to live independently, to hold jobs, and to lead satisfying lives. When society adopts a myth as fact it can do great damage. Myths tend to emphasize limitations, weaknesses, and negative attributes. As a result the self-esteem of the individual will most certainly suffer.

Discrimination and prejudice by the nondisabled can also create feelings of low self-esteem. We live in a society where conformity is stressed and there is little tolerance for individual differences. People with disabilities are a disfavored minority. They are feared, avoided, pitied, and viewed as "strange" and "different." This disability phobia creates a lack of communication and interaction between the disabled and nondisabled. Fortunately there are programs like Special Olympics"and the People First organization, but we have a long way to go. Like the Civil Rights movement of the Sixties, we need a similar effort to more effectively integrate persons with developmental disabilities into the mainstream of our society.

Labeling and Devaluation

Following a five-week hospital stay for a spinal cord injury, the first author was discharged to a rehabilitation facility. My first day there I would realize I was no longer a "regular person." The nurses scurried into my room and announced (as if I weren't there), "Let's get that new quad over to physical therapy." After arriving in physical therapy I heard, "Let's get that new quad down on the mat." Later in group counseling I was told, "Quads can gain independence by . . . " and "Quads need to accept their disability because . . . " I no longer had "person status;" I was now a "quad." To this day I still hate the word. It is dehumanizing. And like so many labels it is imprecise and does not consider the whole person.

For years children with retardation have been classified into an "educable" or "trainable" group based on a hairline I.Q. of 50. No scientific evidence supports this classification process and yet it continues year after year. In addition, results on intelligence tests are dependent on how the subject is feeling on a particular day in a particular testing environment. Labels have the power to shape images and determine major decisions. They can also greatly devalue and depersonalize people when used inappropriately or unwisely.

Lack of Adequate Mental Health Counseling and Services

Counseling by trained mental health professionals is essential to the psychological and social well-being of persons with developmental disabilities and their families. It can be extremely helpful in terms of their emotional needs, their ability to make important decisions, and in connecting them to appropriate community resources. Such counseling was considered impractical and useless up until the early 1950s. The developmentally disabled were thought to be incapable of any significant behavior change, self-understanding or insight. In the 1960s efforts at developing specialized counseling techniques were increased and favorable outcomes occurred in children with developmental disabilities. Since then the quality and quantity of services has increased but unfortunately counselor attitudes toward persons with developmental disabilities still reflect those of the public at large. Most mental health professionals regard them as uninteresting or unworthy of serious consideration. They are reluctant to accept the challenge of working with individuals who may have short attention spans or difficulty in formulating concepts. The authors have done psychological counseling

14

with persons with developmental disabilities and have found them to be refreshingly honest, sincere and significantly free of the "smokescreens" and defenses found with nondisabled clients. An emphasis on issues such as impulse control, frustration tolerance, and problem-solving skills can very positively influence the formation of healthy self-esteem. Mental health professionals should be made aware of the rewards of counseling with persons with developmental disabilities as well as of the extreme need for such therapy.

Chapter III

THE FOUNDATIONS OF SELF-ESTEEM

Self-esteem is like many other terms in counseling and psychology: there is little agreement on its specific definition. For the purposes of this book the definition offered at the beginning of Chapter One will be adequate: *the capacity to view oneself with a fundamental sense of value and competence.* Nathaniel Branden is an author and psychologist who has written extensively on the subject of self-esteem. In his book, *The Psychology of Self-Esteem* (1969, p. 110), he defines self-esteem in this way:

> "Self-esteem has two interrelated aspects: it entails a sense of personal efficacy and a sense of personal worth. It is the integrated sum of self-confidence and self-respect. It is the conviction that one is competent to live and worthy of living."

This corresponds well with our definition and also provides us with a framework for conceptualizing self-esteem building for individuals with developmental disabilities. Self-esteem is basically a combination of *self-confidence* and *self-respect*. We will begin by focusing on the separate components of self-confidence and self-respect. Following this, in Parts Two and Three, we will outline specific strategies for enhancing both in persons with developmental disabilities.

Self-Confidence

Self-confidence involves three interrelated aspects; *action*, *risk-taking* and *control*.

Action in this sense is the ability to respond to life actively rather than passively. It is setting goals and following through on those goals in a decisive, purposeful way. We simply feel better about ourselves when we accomplish things. This can be especially true when it involves something we dislike doing. For many, it is taking the garbage out, mowing the lawn, or getting up when the alarm clock goes off. Despite disliking the task, we've acted, we see results and our self-confidence is strengthened. And then there are the times when we really push or challenge ourselves—that last mile of a marathon, the final hour of a long, hard double shift at work. These experiences reveal our character and expose what we're really "made of." We reach deep down inside ourselves and bring that inner core of strength to the surface. Runners call it "digging down."

For persons with developmental disabilities the act of "digging down" is no different. It may mean added determination in learning a difficult or complex independent living skill. It could involve assertively voicing one's opinion in order to have a building made more accessible or a law made fair. Or it could involve extra effort on the job, often in order to compete with someone who has no disability. Individuals with developmental disabilities must learn to face such challenges in an active, aggressive way. But, more importantly, this "super-active orientation" must become a life philosophy. It is essential to overcoming helplessness, apathy, and discrimination. And because one learns to act directly, one gains control; and self-confidence is strengthened.

Self-confidence is also enhanced through risk-taking. We cannot grow without taking risks. Imagine what life would be like if we never took risks. We would never have taken our first steps as infants, gone out on our first date, or even moved away from home. Normal growth and development would be impossible. But risking is fearful. To risk is to loosen our grip on the safe and familiar and to reach out for something that is uncertain and untested. It may involve giving up certain beliefs, attachments, and allegiances. Because of this, behind every risk is some degree of loss. In making new friends we must sometimes give up past relationships. And in forming new beliefs we must at times abandon old opinions. Because people are frightened by the possibility of loss they often avoid taking any kind of risk. As a result they continually miss out on new experiences and their world becomes very small and their thinking very rigid. Such persons are left feeling isolated, directionless, and insecure.

Risk-taking is crucial for individuals with developmental disabilities. Without risking, isolation from the mainstream of society is a virtual certainty. Without risking, friendships with peers and with the nondisabled becomes extremely difficult. And without risking, gainful employment and independent living can only be an unfulfilled dream. Persons with developmental disabilities must be given opportunities to try out certain risk-taking behaviors in safe and structured settings. Role playing, social skills training, and vocational programs help to provide such opportunities. These options along with specific risk-taking strategies can be quite effective. In Chapter Eight we will discuss the concept of "positive risking" as a technique for confidence-building.

A sense of *control* is the third component essential to healthy self-confidence. We feel better about ourselves when we are in control. We take great pleasure in saying our weight is "under control." In tense or stressful situations we take pride in saying we "maintained control." A sense of control gives us feelings of personal effectiveness and self-discipline. we feel empowered by the belief that we can significantly influence circumstances in our lives. Life is most painful when we feel we are losing control: our job is phased out, we lose a loved one, or we are diagnosed with a serious illness. Suddenly, our sense of control becomes an illusion and we must confront the reality that many circumstances are beyond our influence. But control is crucial to self-confidence. When we feel a sense of control over our lives we act more reasonably and responsibly. We establish specific goals and objectives. And we think more about how our decisions and actions impact those around us.

For persons with developmental disabilities, control over one's environment and one's own self-control are of critical importance for self-confidence. Unfortunately, decision-making and the ability to influence one's circumstances are often taken away from individuals with developmental disabilities. Without being given options, they are often told what to eat, where to live, and who to associate with. Their opinions and feelings are rarely considered. Clearly, children and adults with developmental disabilities do require guidance but, whenever possible, they should be allowed to make decisions and choices for themselves. In this way their feelings of independence, autonomy, and personal control are enhanced.

Self-control is also essential for good self-confidence. It is an extremely important factor in social acceptance, vocational success, and personal growth. A youngster with a developmental disability who can control his feelings and express them appropriately also feels better about himself as a person. His relationships with others will be much more positive and enriching. Teachers and professionals can help persons wtih developmental disabilities learn self-control by placing limits on excessive emotional outbursts, teaching alternative methods for expressing themselves, and by being role models of self-discipline.

Self-Respect

Self-respect, a sense of personal worth, is the other component of self-esteem. It is derived from our values and morals as well as from our feelings of being special and unique. The following little poem really captures the essence of self-respect:

> Knowing the good: we have done it.
> Seeing the beautiful: we have served it.
> Knowing the truth: we have spoken it.

Self-respect involves the three interrelated aspects of *uniqueness*, *connectiveness*, and *integrity*.

A *sense of uniqueness* has to do with how we feel about our own special attributes or characteristics. People with stable, secure self-respect celebrate their uniqueness and individuality. They are proud to be different and love to be labeled "non-comformist." They may cultivate special talents or abilities, trace their heritage or place of origin, or do something unusual with their personal appearance: anything to emphasize their own originality. They recognize that self-respect is closely linked to an individual's sense of uniqueness.

For the individual with a developmental disability a sense of uniqueness can be a crucial factor in developing self-respect. We all need acceptance and approval for what we feel is special about ourselves. Unfortunately, there are many stresses associated with being "different" or "special" in our society, especially if one has a disability. We respect individuality, as long as it does not conflict with our standards of normalcy. And we value originality, providing it doesn't depart too far from our own experience.

The uniqueness associated with having a disability can be a negative experience for many individuals. It is especially important for teachers and professionals to make a special effort in pointing out the strengths and qualities of those with developmental disabilities. Self-respect is basically a result of feeling special in positive ways. We confirm that we are special when others whom we respect support and encourage our abilities. Other ways to develop uniqueness in persons with developmental disabilities include the following:

1. Support them in cultivating unique talents or abilities (artistic, singing, sports).

2. Help them to make the most of their personal appearance (emphasize strengths, downplay weaknesses).

3. Assist them in developing special hobbies or interests (gardening, collecting, camping, scouting).

4. Help them to learn more about their heritage or place of origin (this encourages feelings of individuality).

5. Encourage them to respect themselves (help them to value their own opinions and perceptions).

The second aspect of self-respect is *connectiveness* and it involves how we relate, identify, and "connect" with others. A positive sense of connectiveness is characterized by successful relationships and feelings of belonging. With successful relationships we experience warmth and caring from those who are important to us. This enhances self-respect because when others care about us we naturally feel better about ourselves. Feelings of belonging stem from the sense that we are a part of something. Being a functional and contributing member of a group such as a family, neighborhood, or community provides connectiveness and maximizes self-respect.

Connectiveness is equally important for individuals with developmental disabilities. Unfortunately their sense of connectiveness can be greatly diminished by a lack of stable friendships, family conflicts, and societal prejudice. Teachers and professionals must work especially hard to assist them in forming positive and satisfying relationships (see Chapter Eleven on meaningful relationships). Special attention should also be paid to creating a sense of belonging. Involvement in groups like Boy Scouts, Brownies, Hi-Y, and the People First organization (a self-advocacy group for people with developmental disabilities) can be extremely helpful. With such involvement participants often receive t-shirts or emblems which symbolize their membership and give them a sense of group identity that is concrete and specific. Neighborhood and community activities that are not necessarily disability-oriented (Girl Scouts, Boys' Club, church groups, and volunteer work to help the elderly) can be a positive, connective experience. Feelings of connectiveness can also be derived from exploring one's heritage and past (as was mentioned in the section on uniqueness). Acknowledging one's "roots" (making a family tree, a picture book of relatives, or map of where the family lives) can increase feelings of connectiveness with the past and deepen a sense of belonging in the present.

The third aspect of healthy self-respect is *integrity*. Integrity involves moral and ethical soundness, honesty, and adherence to values. We have integrity when our behavior is in harmony with our professed values. We lose integrity and self-respect when our behavior conflicts with what we believe is right and appropriate. Our values are the criteria by which we judge whether something is right or appropriate. Values also determine attitudes and opinions and are basic to our thoughts and feelings about specific issues, events, and relationships. Values must be clearly defined and adhered to in order to maintain a high level of integrity and self-respect.

A strong sense of integrity is no less important for persons with developmental disabilities. Integrity and values provide a much needed framework for appropriate behavior at work, in public, and in sexual situations. Unfortunately, it is thought that impaired cognitive abilities lead to little or no capacity for moral decision-making. But this is a false assumption. A group of studies by Stephens and her colleagues (Mahoney and Stephens, 1974; McLaughlin and Stephens, 1974; Moore and Stephens, 1974; Stephens and McLaughlin, 1974) have suggested that individuals with developmental disabilities do improve over time on tests of moral judgment and conduct. Values are most often learned through modeling. If teachers and professionals exemplify adherence to good moral conduct in their own lives, then children and adults with developmental disabilities will be more inclined to model such behavior. In addition, value clarification exercises can be helpful in enhancing self-respect and integrity. See Chapter Twelve for an expanded discussion.

Part II

Strategies for Promoting Self-Confidence

Chapter IV

NURTURE SUCCESS

We've all heard the saying "Nothing succeeds like success." It could also be said that nothing builds self-confidence like success. In fact, virtually all the strategies in this book for increasing self-esteem are also meant to promote the experience of success. People with high self-esteem have almost always met with some degree of success. By success we do not mean owning half a dozen Rolls-Royces or a 40-foot yacht. Instead we refer to the experience of having satisfying relationships, fufilling work, and a sense of purpose in life. Our definition is more closely linked to something Will Rogers once said: "In order to succeed, you must know what you are doing, like what you are doing, and believe in what you are doing."

Success doesn't come easily to persons with developmental disabilities. Too often their abilities and potential have been underestimated or overlooked. Or they're simply not given a chance to succeed because of a label that was attached to them early in their lives. But that doesn't mean it's too late. The experience of success can begin the process of reversing a negative self-image. The following guidelines may be helpful in promoting success with children and adults with developmental disabilities:

1. Allow the individual to choose the new skill or ability to be worked on.
    Rather than choosing for her, follow her lead, and support what she wants to do. Watch for sparks of interest and use whatever motivation is present. Often that interest will provide the way to a succesful learning experience.

2. Use all available information about the person to assist him.
    Talk to former teachers, his parents, the staff at the group home or vocational program, anyone who has had contact with him and knows how he learns and what motivates him. Using this information, start the person out at his current success level instead of "reinventing the wheel."

3. Keep expectations realistic.

   What seems practical and reasonable to you may not be to her. Having expectations that are too high promotes failure rather than success. Check out how she's feeling about a certain task. It shows her that you respect her opinions.

4. Acknowledge successes.

   We are products of an educational system that has traditionally emphasized what is done wrong instead of what is done right. Testing procedures highlight negative evaluations because what gets marked and noticed are the wrong answers. We are evaluated in light of our failures instead of validated for what we do correctly. In working with persons with developmental disabilities the teacher or professional should be careful to focus on the positive by pointing out progress and improvements. Keeping a record or chart is helpful to show when and where growth has occurred. Reviewing it with the individual will also reinforce continued success.

5.	Utilize existing successes.
	Take advantage of what they already have going for
	them. Capitalize on successes that already exist. For
	example, at the group home where she lives, Cindy
	was continually being complimented for the way she
	set the dinner table. Everything was always very neat
	and orderly and often she would add special touches
	like flowers or decorative napkins. Cindy had already
	demonstrated success in this area and she felt good
	about herself for it. With some help in working on
	appropriate social behavior, Cindy was able to get a
	job in a hotel restaurant setting up tables for large
	dinners and conventions. She loves the job and her
	self-confidence has increased dramatically. As
	Cindy's story points out, success builds most easily
	and effectively on past successes.

6.	Recognize that the process is most important.
	It is the process and not necessarily the outcome or
	attained goal that nurtures success and builds self-
	confidence. Break tasks down into small steps and
	avoid needless failure whenever possible. In giving
	feedback provide continual support and
	encouragement. Working and practicing to be

especially good at a skill or hobby also creates a special feeling of success.

For example, there is Roy's story. All those at the vocational program knew Roy was very well coordinated. He could lift and carry things of varying size and weight better than anybody. Roy also liked bowling. Every Saturday afternoon he would watch it on TV, but he had never actually tried it. He was scared of being laughed at. A staff person named Doug at Roy's job site heard about Roy's interest in bowling. Doug was something of an accomplished bowler himself, having bowled in a league for a number of years. Although Roy was scared, Doug convinced him to try bowling just one time. The two went on a night when there weren't many people at the alley. Roy's first few attempts were "gutter balls." He felt like quitting right then and there. But Doug showed him the proper form and was very patient. Soon Roy was rolling the ball right down the middle of the lane and even hit a strike. After that Doug and Roy bowled every Thursday night for almost a year. Roy practiced very hard and never gave up in his efforts to keep improving his score. Currently Roy is bowling in a league and his average is 150! Roy derives a special feeling of success from his bowling and this feeling helps him to succeed in other areas of his life as well.

In the book *100 Ways to Enhance Self-Concept in the Classroom* by Jack Canfield and Harold C. Wells, there is a group exercise entitled "Success Sharing." Students are asked to share a success or accomplishment during a recent period of time, the past week, the last month, over the weekend, etc. The teacher or professional may have to prod those persons with especially low self-concepts to come up with something. Using special knowledge about group members he could ask questions such as, "Did you finish the chores assigned to you at home?" or "How did you do in the Special Olympics recently?" or "What did you accomplish at the vocational training program last week?" These certainly don't have to be large accomplishments, just things they feel good about. Keeping a record of these successes and then reviewing occasionally would be helpful too. The important thing is that the students begin to focus on the positive aspects of themselves.

As a child David (a young person with Down syndrome) wanted badly to be successful like his twin brother who was athletic, well-coordinated and quick. David's mother realized that she would have to nurture this success and that she would have to support activities and hobbies different from David's twin or he would always come out on the short end of the competition. She also looked for hobbies and interests also that could follow David into adulthood, knowing how long it might take for him to be successful.

Swimming was one of his first successes, nurtured by private lessons, lots of practice and the knowledge that this success could lead to a lifetime of good health. It was something he could do alone or with others.

A ping pong table at the swim center caught David's eye one day and so his mother seized the opportunity when he was twelve to nurture a hobby, skill and success that has become a lifetime interest and a source of friendship sharing now that he is an adult.

Chapter V

DEVELOP INDEPENDENCE AND AUTONOMY

There's an old Chinese proverb that goes, "If you give a man a fish, you feed him for the day; but if you teach him how to fish, you feed him for life." Assisting others to be independent and self-sufficient helps them to carry out a very basic instinctual need. From the moment we are born we begin striving for independence. We desire separateness from our parents in order to capture feelings of autonomy and self-reliance. In the teen-age years, separateness may turn to rebellion as we attempt to declare our independence and maturity. The need for indepenence also reflects a need for self-esteem. As we gain independence, we acquire confidence, control, and a healthy self-appraisal.

For persons with developmental disabilities, independence is the foundation on which to build self-confidence. When maximized, independence provides feelings of success, accomplishment and empowerment. Being able to say, "I'm living on my own," or "I did it by myself" gives an individual with a disability a tremendous amount of pride. There is no greater gift a teacher or professional can give than that of independence or autonomy. As the philosopher Soren Kierkegaard once said: "The most one human being can do for another is to help him stand on his own two feet—alone." But independence is not easily taught. Often children and adolescents with developmental disabilities are overprotected or isolated. They are not given the opportunity to develop habits of exploration or self-reliance. This makes the job of teaching or encouraging independence much more difficult. Acting independently has a variety of meanings for persons with a developmental disability. For some it can mean tying their own shoes while for others it involves living by themselves or getting married. The following guidelines for promoting independence will need to be adapted according to the individual's specific circumstances.

1.   Encourage them to make choices.
Too often, persons with developmental disabilities are not given choices. They are told what to do, where to live, and who to have as friends. Their feelings and ideas are thought to have little value. Involving them in choosing

builds trust in their ability to exercise their own will and make decisions. It gives them a sense of control over their lives as well as a feeling that their opinions really matter. Also, with experience in decision-making they don't feel as helpless when faced with new situations or challenges. This is especially helpful in terms of the challenges they will face in learning to be independent.

2.   Help them to deal with frustration.
In learning new skills to become independent, frustration is inevitable. And because of their disability, frustration is likely to be a constant companion throughout their lives. If frustration becomes excessive, a "timeout" period away from the new task or skill may be required. The old idea of counting to ten along with slow and rhythmic deep breathing may also be helpful. Then with support and encouragement, help them to work through the problem or difficulty. Give suggestions and advise if you need to but basically let them solve the problem. A sense of humor is also a valuable tool for dealing with frustration. Life is too short to be taken so seriously. Together with them, laugh and joke about the problem; you'll find that it will renew your energy and enthusiasm to solve it.

3.   Allow them to make mistakes.

It is hard at times to resist intervening in order to prevent a mistake from being made. You want them to learn to do things right and be the best they can be. But by not stepping in to correct them continually you are showing you accept them. And acceptance by others, especially those in authority, is important to self-esteem. You are also showing them that they don't have to be perfect, that they can make mistakes and fail, without losing self-esteem.

4.   Stimulate them with challenges.

Challenges develop skills and abilities and help them feel they are capable and competent. Make sure the challenge is difficult enough so it does stretch their abilities but not so hard that they will be reluctant to try. Let them help choose the challenge so it will be something they are interested in. Also, steer them in the direction of an area where they have already shown some ability.

5.   Provide role models who can demonstrate
       independence.

There is nothing quite as motivating as seeing another individual with a disability similar to your own demonstrating independence. For many people with disabilities it is a matter of pride and self-respect to show that they can be as independent as the next person. For the person with a developmental disability, seeing or talking with someone living independently in an apartment, in a group home, or performing any number of independent living skills could be invaluable incentive to get them started on their own path to increased independence.

6. Enlist the help of those who come in contact with the person.

The encouragement and support of a wide variety of people can greatly aid others in their attempts to be more independent. Vocational instructors, counselors, cooks, housekeepers, physical therapists, family members, can all serve as motivators for increased independence. They can inquire as to how their progress is coming, what their latest hurdle has been, and how they might assist. As a result these persons are more motivated to work because they are continually reporting to others. Most people do not like to appear as though they have been "sloughing off."

When Pam was four years old, her parents were overwhelmed with her dependence. While Pam was a very delightful child, her developmental disability required lots of parental prompting, cueing, and reinforcement for her to learn. Her parents remembered that her older brothers at this age were able to be independent in many activities; in fact the boys emphatically insisted on dressing themselves, walking without holding hands, etc. It seemed as though autonomy and independence happened without parental intervention.

With guidance from a Pilot parent, Pam's parents began structuring time for Pam to be alone in her room to listen to her cassette tapes, look at books and play with favorite toys. These times were brief yet unsupervised. Dressing was a slow training process but as Pam acquired a new skill, her parents gradually removed their help. Mom set out Pam's clothes and left her to put them on unassisted with the encouraging words: "Pam, I know you can dress yourself. Mommy will be back in fifteen minutes to help you with your shoes." The pride and praise of her parents helped Pam take greater steps to independence. Family and staff intermittently praised her for her progress and soon Pam learned the connection between her own actions—playing quietly alone for an hour) and the results—praise and quality time with parents and family.

Candy needed help initially in weight control. When she first moved to the group home, staff developed a fitness plan and carefully monitored her food intake. Once she learned her exercise program, they turned the responsibility of doing it daily over to Candy. A chart was made to record her exercises (a self reinforcer and motivator). Soon Candy got the connection between her exercising and eating habits and her loss of weight. Family, staff and group home workers praised her but they gave her self-responsibility and independence. Later she used this self-reliance and autonomy to reach out for friendship and attain other goals.

Chapter VI

COMMUNICATE ASSERTIVELY

In living and communicating with others, we behave in many different ways. Sometimes we fail to speak up, draw lines, set limits, or say no to people and demands. This difficulty can lead to procrastination, powerlessness, low self-esteem and feelings of being "walked over" or "stepped on." When we cannot refuse the requests of others we live our lives according to their priorities rather than our own. We suffer in silence and accumulate resentment, bitterness, and anger. Sometime we feel that the only way to get our needs met is to be demanding and fight for our rights. We blame, threaten, humiliate, and almost always step on the personal rights of others. Afterwards we end up feeling guilty and lonely.

There is a way of expressing ourselves, getting our needs met, and defending ourselves, without being passive or aggressive. To be assertive means to stand up for personal rights, beliefs, and feelings in direct and honest ways. It also means respecting the needs, feelings and rights of other people. In addition, assertiveness positively influences self-confidence and self-respect.

1. Assertion gives a greater sense of control over our lives because as we stand up for ourselves in honest, responsible ways, we are more likely to get our needs met.

2. Because assertiveness eventually results in improved self-confidence we reduce the need for the approval of others and can feel more secure within ourselves.

3. Assertive behavior enhances self-respect because we do not compromise our integrity or values.

4. We gain respect for others because we have the courage to take a stand, and deal with problems in open and honest ways.

5. With assertion, rather than aggression, we have the capacity to create more satisfying relationships because we are more willing to talk things out in a constructive, honest manner, and with better

relationships our sense of connectiveness is enhanced and self-respect improves.

Assertiveness training is especially important for children or adults with developmental disabilities. Besides being an invaluable tool for effectively dealing with sexual exploitation, assertion skills also help in overcoming feelings of powerlessness, helplessness, and diminished self-confidence. In addition, because persons with developmental disabilities were often overprotected or isolated in childhood, they may be lacking in the social skills needed to combat shyness, loneliness and prejudice from the nondisabled. Assertion training can be an excellent first step in dealing with such issues.

The authors have found that generally group assertion training is most effective for individuals with developmental disabilities, although individual training does have the advantage of creating a safer environment for those who are fearful of group interaction. It also allows the trainer to teach immediate assertion skills for those who may be in crisis situations. Still, group assertion training does provide certain advantages:

1.   Individuals can bring real life assertion problems to the group and role play with one another.

2.   During group sessions participants engage in nonassertive and aggressive behaviors which can be identified and worked on.

3.   Group members can support and encourage each other's attempts at assertion skills.

4.   Assertion skills can be strengthened through modeling the behavior of the trainer and participants.

The first step in beginning the group is to clearly explain the difference between passive, assertive, and aggressive. The chart below provides some examples, but the teacher or professional will need to tailor them to the intellectual functioning of the group. For better group understanding, it is possible that the terms passive, assertive, and aggressive may have to be changed to adjectives like lazy, honest, or demanding, or to descriptors such as "wimpy" or "pushy." It is very important to use humor whenever possible and make the experience fun. Overacting, exaggerating, and/or role-playing with another staff person can be helpful and can emphasize the differences in communication styles.

After going over the different types of communication, the Assertion Quiz below can help to determine how much was learned. Again, humor and exaggeration in the presentation and discussion of the items on the quiz can be important in reinforcing concepts. When the differences between passive, aggressive, and assertive seem fairly adequately understood, it may be time to ask the participants if they have any real life situations where they feel a need to be more assertive. The group members may choose either the trainer or another group member to role play with. It is not unusual that group members will be shy about volunteering a situation so the trainer should be ready with several practice role plays. These could involve any number of people (a staff person, teacher, peer) or situations (conflict at the group home, dispute at work, problem with parents). If trainers have access to the equipment, videotaping can enhance and reinforce the learning process. Participants can observe themselves and refine and improve on their newly acquired skills. Videotapes can be saved and then shown in subsequent sessions to illustrate progress. Also, playing back only the video portion (no sound) can sometimes be a valuable source of feedback on nonverbal behaviors.

Much more could be said about assertiveness and persons with developmental disabilities. In this book we have chosen to discuss a variety of techniques to raise self-esteem, so we have limited ourselves to only discussing the basics of assertion training. Because of the importance of assertiveness, teachers and professionals may want to look into some of the mainstream assertion books (see reference list in back of book) and then tailor the ideas and strategies to the individuals they are working with.

ASSERTION QUIZ

Instructions: This quiz contains ten interpersonal situations with responses that are passive, assertive, or aggressive. Read each situation and response carefully then indicate in the right hand column which communication style is being used. The answers appear at the end of the quiz.

Situation	Response	Passive, Assertive, or Aggressive
1. You're in a restaurant and the waiter brings you a steak that is rare instead of well done as you ordered it. You respond,	You're crazy if you think I'm going to eat this lousy steak!	_____
2. You've been talking on the phone for a long time with a friend and you'd like the conversation to end. You say,	Excuse me, I'm really sorry, there's someone at my door. I hope you don't mind. I need to hang up.	_____
3. Someone in the neighborhood where you live offers you drugs. You respond,	No, I don't use drugs.	_____
4. You've enjoyed the way your teacher has taught a class. You say,	Thank you for making this class so interesting.	_____
5. You've been looking forward to watching a special TV program all week long. Just as you sit down to watch, someone comes in and turns the channel to another show. You say,	All right, all right, that's it! If you don't turn that channel back to my program I'm gonna punch you right in the nose!	_____

6. Someone touches you in a place where you don't want to be touched. You say,

No. Don't do that. I don't want you to touch me at all.

_____

7. Your roommate is always leaving your room in a mess. You say,

I think it's about time you stopped leaving this room in such a mess. Clean it up now!

_____

8. A loud stereo upstairs is disturbing you. You go upstairs to talk to the person and say,

Hi, I live downstairs. Your stereo is loud and is bothering me. Would you please turn it down?

_____

9. A friend wants to borrow your new hat hat. It looks like it might rain. You respond,

Well . . . I guess that would be okay. I sure hope it doesn't rain.

_____

10. You're hoping to go someplace special this weekend. You think to yourself,

Gee, I sure hope that someone will ask me to go someplace this weekend.

_____

Answers:

1.	Aggressive		6.	Assertive
2.	Passive		7.	Aggressive
3.	Assertive		8.	Assertive
4.	Assertive		9.	Passive
5.	Aggressive		10.	Passive

Penny's mom's greatest fear as Penny developed was that she might one day be a victim of physical or sexual exploitation. As a single parent, Mom tended to be overprotective. As Penny moved towards her teens, Mom began exploring sterilization. Her research showed Mom that sterilization was not the answer to exploitation (it would not make Penny less vulnerable to unwanted approaches) but that basic assertion skills and effective decision making skills must be paramount. Mom started teaching Penny choice-making. Laying out several choices of outfits to choose from to wear each day, allowing Penny to make selections for family activities and favorite meals—both were beginning steps to choice making. Mom learned too that even persons with developmental disabilities have the right to express "likes" and "dislikes" and that expressing these are important protective skills.

Too often persons with developmental disabilities are taught to be compliant, to follow orders without using their own decision-making abilities. This situation makes life easy for parents and professionals but sets up the person with disabilities for exploitation. Basic assertion skills include having the right to say "no" to teachers, parents, and other persons. It means expressing your own "likes" and "dislikes" and having your differences valued. Young adults hungry to please others lack the self-confidence to say "no" to exploitation.

Chapter VII

SET GOALS AND OBJECTIVES

If we really want to take an active role in satisfying the needs and desires in our lives, then we must have goals. Once we have goals then we can devise a plan or blueprint for action. We can break down the steps of getting us from where we are now to where we want to be. Some other reasons for setting goals are as follows:

1. Goals provide an opportunity for evaluating accomplishments and discussing problems.

2. Goals give us a standard against which progress can be evaluated.

3. Goals provide direction and motivation.

4. Goals help us to gain perspective on how short term efforts and long range plans are related.

6. Goals provide a foundation for setting new goals— they help us to keep reaching out.

Basically, goals give purpose and meaning to our lives. They give us something to aim for and achieve. Achieving what we want out of life is like climbing to the top of a ladder. We don't leap to the top of the ladder, we have to take a few steps at a time. Our plan for achieving what we want out of life must have steps too. Otherwise, we will be unable to climb. And as each step of the ladder is achieved, our self-confidence progressively gets stronger.

Goals serve a similar function for persons with developmental disabilities. As goals are set and achieved in areas like independent living, social gains, or vocational pursuits, self-confidence is increasingly enhanced. It is especially important to emphasize goals that are achievable and realistic. Otherwise we may be setting people up for needless failure and frustration. But this is often a difficult judgment to make. The authors have been impressed many times by persons wtih developmental disabilities who, after being told that they have certain insurmountable limitations, march out and overcome those limitations (see the story of Tim at the end of the chapter). But at times, goals or dreams do fall within the realm of fantasy, such as wishes to become brain surgeons or astronauts. It is best to

54

help a child or adult with a developmental disability focus on hopeful yet realistic possibilities. They should be encouraged to "stretch" their capabilities but not strive for something that is clearly and totally out of reach.

Role models can be instrumental in providing the motivation to set goals. The first author recalls an incident in the adjustment to his own spinal cord injury. It was approximately a year since my diving accident and I was not getting any sensation or movement back. I was feeling increasingly hopeless and depressed, devoid of any meaning or sense of direction in my life. Sensing this, my father learned of a young woman who was in similar circumstances but who had begun to turn her life around. He invited her to come over and visit me. Her name was Sherry and she drove up in a modified van with a wheelchair lift. Besides driving, Sherry was also attending college classes, dating, and living in an apartment with a roommate. Sherry gave me new hope that, although disabled, I could still live a satisfying and meaningful life. I began to set goals based on Sherry's successes, as well as my own interests and abilities.

Role models don't necessarily have to be disabled to inspire persons with disabilities to set goals. Attention may also be directed to the achievable qualities in role models who are not disabled. For example, if a tennis player is admired by a young girl with cerebral palsy, the child could be encouraged to focus on qualities such as commitment to the sport, fair play, and self-discipline, rather than focusing solely on the person's athletic abilities. Similarly, if a young man with a developmental disability wants to be a politician or president he could be guided to develop his own leadership abilities (decision-making, giving speeches, etc.) for use at school, in a group home, or in special clubs or organizations.

In the book *100 Ways to Enhance Self-Concept in the Classroom* , there is a self-esteem enhancing exercise entitled "I Want To Be." It asks that students choose a person they admire very much. It may be a person historical, fictional, living or dead. They are asked why they chose that person. What qualities does that person possess? Why is he or she to be admired? Then the student is asked to compare themselves to the person they have chosen to emulate. What would they have to do to be more like that person? What changes would they have to make?

How could they go about making them? The students then set personal goals for achieving these desired changes.

The authors have had success in using this exercise in group work with persons with developmental disabilities. A young man named Mark selected the professional wrestler Hulk Hogan as the person he admired most. According to Mark, Hulk Hogan is strong and is one of the "good guy" wrestlers. Mark then set a goal of exercising more often and of playing more fairly in sporting activities with his friends. Another participant in the group named Jill chose the country singer Loretta Lynn. Jill admired Loretta Lynn for her singing abilities and set a goal to improve her own singing enough so that she could sing in her church choir. Bill, a third group member, chose his mother because she is very sweet and loving. His goal was to begin treating others in more loving ways.

Goal-setting should be a cooperative planning process between the teacher or professional and the person with a developmental disability. If the individual has a voice in determining and setting goals, then his motivation and enthusiasm will stay high. He will also feel more value as a person because his opinions are being considered. Other guidelines for effective goal setting are as follows:

1. Goals need to be specific and written down. Progress can only be made when goals are clearly defined. Example: "Craig will work at the community sheltered workshop and do electronics assembly work parttime in the mornings from 8:00 a.m. to noon." Also, once a goal is written down it actually becomes a goal; it is no longer simply a wish.

2. Goals should contain specific time deadlines. Arriving at target dates for completing each step of a plan provides constant reinforcement and a sense of acomplishment that helps sustain motivation. Example: Craig will begin work on November 1 and will work until December 20.

3. Goals should be broken down into objectives. Goals are long term outcomes. Objectives are measurable results within short time frames. Objectives provide real feelings of accomplishment. An example of Craig's objectives include: (1) to put away five dollars per week to save up for Christmas presents; (2) to be

on time to work each day; and (3) to ride public transportation once a week.

4.   Goals and objectives should be reviewed often to check progress. It is very reinforcing to discover we are meeting our objectives and accomplishing our goals. Craig's self-confidence will grow each step of the way that his objectives are being realized.

Assisting persons with developmental disabilities to set goals greatly helps them to build self-confidence. Goals give them a much needed sense of direction and purpose.

Tim's parents have been teaching him about goal setting almost from the moment he was born. Wanting him to learn to walk, his mom encouraged him to creep by putting Tim on the floor with his favorite toys just out of reach. By age 2 1/2 he had learned to walk. They set a new goal of talking as mom and dad encouraged sounds, reinfored early attempts, and finally heard sentences. Little League baseball, Cub Scouts, and public school were goals set forth by this joyful young man with Down syndrome. Nurtured by the support and encouragement of his parents, Tim met with success. And NOTHING SUCCEEDS LIKE SUCCESS. So as Tim moved on to junior high and high school, new goals appeared: riding the school bus with the "regular kids," managing the ball team, having a job, becoming an Eagle Scout, owning his own business and living on his own.

Today each of these goals has been met. In 1985, after 21 badges were completed, Tim accomplished his final community service project for becoming an Eagle Scout by giving over 25 "Disability Awareness" talks to his classmates, schoolchildren, parents, professionals and civic club members: "My name is Tim . . . I was born with Down syndrome . . . I would like to tell you how it feels to be retarded . . . how it feels to have people make fun of you . . . ." Tim gives his audiences something to think about.

At age 22 Tim has met more goals than some do in a lifetime. He's contributed to the understanding of many with disabilities, he's started his own "Farm Fresh Eggs" business tending to his brood of chickens, has completed high school, held many part-time jobs, learned to ride an off-road vehicle, cares for countless pets, and lives on his own in an apartment with minimal help.

Tim's got a lot more goals set for himself. They include girls, travel and more money in his pocket.

Chapter VIII

PRACTICE POSITIVE-RISKING

It is interesting that the word "risk" has only negative connotations in our language. The dictionary defines it as a "hazard; peril; exposure to loss or injury." We typically associate a risk with something dangerous or fearful. And yet without risk there would be no progress or personal growth. We must risk in order to accomplish and succeed. But risking must be tempered by reason and common sense. There are those who take unnecessary, hazardous risks; the individual who drinks and drives, the young person who experiments with dangerous drugs. Such people are often compulsive riskers and have powerful self-destructive urges.

We must look for a balance between taking suicidal chances on the one hand and running from risking on the other. This balance involves carefully evaluating new things we try and asking "What's the risk and what's the potential payoff?" In deciding whether to risk or not we should also ask ourselves "Will I be better off for having taken this risk, even if I don't succeed?" In other words, can something be learned from having gone through the process of risking? Can it positively impact our lives? This is what is meant by "positive risking." The payoff, as well as the process of risking, are both seen as being potentially self-enhancing and positive experiences.

Successful risk-taking is essential in helping persons with developmental disabilities to build self-confidence. They may be fearful of the risks involved in seeking a job, making a new friend, or moving into a group home. If their fears can be reduced, then they can approach the risk with a greater chance of success. The steps involved in positive risking can help persons with developmental disabilities confront fear before the actual risk is taken. In this way they move into the risk with confidence and with feelings of having their "bases covered." The teacher or professional should be aware that not all the steps will be applicable to every situation or set of circumstances. Also, the strategies will need to be tailored to the individual's level of intellectual functioning. Positive risking involves the following steps:

1.   Reinforce efforts to prepare for a risk-taking situation. All too often we focus too much on the goal and not enough on the process it took to get us there. If we don't reach the goal or get the payoff then we feel worthless, our self-respect suffers, and we feel our efforts were in vain. It is important to support efforts made in preparation for the risk. For example, let's say you are working with a young man named Charlie who has a crush on a girl but is terribly afraid to ask her to the specialized recreation dance. You have agreed to help him overcome his fear. First, you and Charlie decide he needs to look his best when he asks her to go so he gets a haircut and buys a new shirt. Then you both work on when he will ask her and what he will say. After each one of these steps you would encourage Charlie's efforts in order to support the process leading up to the risk. This helps to insure that it will be a valuable experience regardless of the actual outcome.

2.   Help them to develop a strategy of working up to the actual risk.
Careful, measured increases in risk are less anxiety producing. For example, when we learn to ride a

bicycle we do not start out in heavy automobile
traffic. Instead, we pick a street where if we fall
down, at least we will not get run over. In Charlie's
case, he could work up to the big risk of asking her
out on a date by first asking her to dance, then
possibly just chatting with her a little while, followed
by asking her to have a soft drink with him. These
gradual increases in risk would also give him a feel
for how receptive she is.

3.   Ask them, "What's the worst thing that can happen?"
This is in reference to the big risk. If they fail or if it
doesn't turn out right, how bad can it really be? Here,
you are essentially asking for a "catastrophe report,"
outlining specifically what the effects might be and
how they might cope with it. Charlie may speculate
that she could laugh at him, call him a "nerd," and
then tell everyone in the vocational program where
they are both employed the whole story. Then you
would help him with a plan to deal with this worst
case scenario. As much as possible you would want
him to come up with his own ideas, but if he is having
difficulties you would make suggestions. For
example, have him tell people in the vocational

program that it's her loss, not his, and that she doesn't know what she's missing. And that she's the "nerd" because she won't have the golden opportunity to go out dancing with him. Preparing for the worst helps them to move into the risk with less anxiety and a greater chance for success.

4. Role play the risk-taking situation.
    Practicing and refining what to say and how to say it can substantially reduce the fear associated with many risks. You could begin by asking Charlie what he might want to say to the young woman in terms of general conversation and "small talk." Offer help with phrasing, showing interest, making eye contact, and being a good listener (see Chapter Eleven). Then role play the situation with Charlie as himself and you as the young woman. Give him feedback as to what he's doing right and what he could improve on. Work on it until Charlie feels comfortable and his lines flow as smoothly and naturally as possible.

5. Ask them to recall past similar experiences.
    Bringing to mind a past similar experience where he demonstrated success can increase the confidence

needed for risk-taking. When we are especially fearful we lose perspective. We can think only of the failures in our past and problems of the present. We often forget that we have performed well in past similar situations. The actual difficulty of a situation and our ability to handle it can best be evaluated by recalling similar past experiences and making a comparison. Even if the situations are not completely alike, there will be aspects that are similar. Charlie may have had past friendships or love relationships that required assertiveness or good communication skills. He could draw on these past experiences to make his present risk-taking situation easier.

Helen Keller once said, "Security is mostly a superstition. It does not exist in nature, nor do the children of men as a whole experience it. Avoiding danger is no safer in the long run than outright exposure. Life is either a daring adventure or nothing." We must risk in order to grow and change. Everything we really want in life involves taking a risk. Risking wakes us up and makes us feel exhilarated and alive.

Frances is a person with cerebral palsy and retardation. When she transitioned to high school, she and her parents were presented with a scary "risk" opportunity—riding public transportation independently. Knowing that Frances often viewed herself through her parents' eyes, they were careful not to discuss their fears in her presence. They didn't want her to internalize a view of herself as helpless. Reviewing the challenge and risk, they decided that without the risk experience, their goal of independence might never be realized for Frances.

They began by reinforcing in Frances her pedestrian travel skills and their pleasure with her safety awareness. They encouraged her by telling her they were confident that with positive practice and coaching she would learn to ride public transportation independently.

Frances's parents worked out a plan for training and "shadowing" Frances to relieve their fears and to give Frances the support that she needed. They pointed out to her that she had been successful in the past at mastering new skills using this approach. She had learned to work in the school cafeteria, to swim and to walk two blocks to a friend's home.

Plans were made for how to handle missed bus stops, late buses, or feeling lost. The trainer (coach) and Frances's parents provided Frances with identification cards, phone numbers and a card with money to make two phone calls.

Many repetitions, many escorted bus rides were taken, as well as practice at bus mix-ups before Frances ever rode the bus "alone" with a shadow following her. In fact she was shadowed for five days. Since she did not make an error in those five days, she was put on an intermittent shadowing check (probe) to see that she was maintaining her bus skills.

A great risk was taken in this bid for independent travel but the gains for Frances were not only bus independence but the joy and pride of taking a challenging risk and succeeding!

Chapter IX

UTILIZE POSITIVE SELF STATEMENTS

We all have a negative inner voice that attacks and judges us. It calls us names, blames us when things go wrong, and tries to convince us we are worthless. This inner voice is our own personal critic. People with poor self-esteem tend to have a more vocal and vicious critic. The critic makes us believe we should be perfect, and then lets us have it when we make the slightest mistake. He keeps a record of our failures and shortcomings, but rarely mentions our successes or strengths. The critic's major assignment is to constantly undermine our self-esteem and self-worth.

The critic began working on us in childhood when we first started receiving negative programming. In his book *What To Say When You Talk to Yourself*, psychologist Shad Helmstetter reports that during the first eighteen years of our lives, if we grew up in a reasonably positive home, we would have been told "No!" or what we could not do, more than 148,000 times. He also explains that behavioral researchers have discovered that seventy-seven percent of everything we say to ouselves is negative or works against us.

For persons with developmental disabilities the critic is probably working overtime. He constantly harrasses them with labels such as stupid, inferior, incompetent, and dumb. And most likely, because of early devaluation and isolation, children and adolescents with developmental disabilities received substantially more than 148,000 negative messages. In comparisons to nondisabled siblings and other "normal" children, they always came up short. All their lives the emphasis has been on their limitations and lack of abilities. For them, thinking and behaving in positive ways has been a continual struggle.

Positive self-talk can be a valuable tool in helping to turn around negative thinking patterns and increase self-confidence. The basic idea is to send our negative internal critic on vacation and replace him with someone who will be affirming and positive. This is done through learning and practicing specific self-statements which are positive and self-enhancing. As the self-statements are read and practiced more and more, they are increasingly internalized and will positively affect our mood, outlook, and degree of self-esteem. Self-statements can also be used to reduce stress. They may include phrases like "I can meet this challenge" or "I will be calm and relaxed." For enhancing self-esteem, statements include "I am a good person," "I am fun to be with," or "I am nice looking." We have also included self-statements in this chapter for motivation and assertiveness. In working with persons with developmental disabilities, the authors have found that positive self-talk can be used with an individual or in a group setting. Individually, more time and attention can be paid toward learning what specific self-statements are most effective. In a group the process of making a self-talk tape can be especially fun and that enthusiasm is reflected in the end product. The following guidelines may be helpful in utilizing positive self-talk:

1. Explain the concept.
   Tell them that inside our heads we all say mean things to ourselves or call ourselves names (stupid, jerk, dummy) and this makes us feel bad. Explain that you're going to come up with some nice things to say to yourselves and then put them on a cassette tape.

2.   Make a list of personalized self-talk that would be most relevant to the individuals in the group. The authors co-led a counseling group for several years with adolescents with cerebral palsy. In utilizing positive self-talk the adolescents found it most effective when they used the language of their own generation: "I'm chilled out," "I'm looking awesome," and "fresh" and "rad."

3.   Make a cassette tape of positive self-statements. This is especially good for slow readers or nonreaders. Have group members take turns reading the statements they've agreed to onto a tape recorder. Pause after each statement and let the tape run in silence for the length of time it took to read the statement. Then, later, the phrase can be repeated aloud when an individual is using the tape. Group members will be shy at first of the tape recorder. Practice ahead of time and assure them they can try as many times as they need to in order to get it right.

4.   Intermix inspirational music onto the tape. This will help insure that they'll actually use the tape as well as reinforce the ideas behind the self-

statements. For example, for self-esteem building try Whitney Houston's "The Greatest Love of All." For motivation — the theme music from the movie "Rocky." For reducing stress — only music that is calming and relaxing.

5. Have them listen to the tape in the morning.
   It's a healthy way to begin the day because it affords an emotional boost. To keep from disturbing others they could listen on a portable tape player with headphones. Also, listening to the self-esteem portion of the tape in front of the mirror can help to improve body image and self-acceptance.

6. Have them combine listening to the tape with visualization.
   This may be difficult for persons with developmental disabilities. Some have trouble concentrating on a single image for short periods. If they can master it have them imagine doing something successfully (giving a speech, working, bowling) while they're listening to the tape. This will strengthen the effectiveness of the self-statements.

7. Have them keep one very special belief in mind when they're listening to the tape.
    They are good, worthy people who are deserving of love and happiness in life. This very important belief will make the self-statements more powerful and long lasting.

Positive self-statements are not a panacea for individuals with developmental disabilities who have poor self-esteem. But along with other strategies, they are a valuable tool for helping people to feel better about themselves by beginning the process of eliminating negative thinking. It should be noted, however, that some people with developmental disabilities who are suffering from low self-esteem or from depression would be best served by seeing their physician or a mental health professional.

Judy had always longed for a place in the spotlight. Then one day it happened. She was elected president of the Oregon PEOPLE FIRST organization, a dream come true for this developmentally disabled young adult after spending fourteen years in a state residential institution. When Judy realized that this new honor would mean public speaking, officiating at meetings and meeting lots of new people, she was afraid.

She was afraid that the cerebral palsy that challenged her speaking would make people think she was stupid, slow and unable to carry out the duties of president. Judy's self-talk was very negative.

One of the helpers caught on to Judy's self-talk and helped her form some new self-talk.
"I can handle this."
"I can be heard."
"I can talk as though only one person is in this room."

The cover of this book shows Judy in her hour of honor addressing over one thousand persons at the annual PEOPLE FIRST convention.

"I can meet this challenge."
And indeed she did!

Data show clearly that how we feel about our chances for success greatly affect that success.

For an older child or teen we might encourage them to say:

"I can meet this challenge."
"I've done it before, I'll do it again."
"I can handle this."

For the child experiencing sadness we might teach him or her to say:

"I will be strong."
"I am not going to let this bother me."

For anger:
"Why am I angry?"
"Being angry won't help."

Being able to express an emotion can also defuse it. When your child expressses anger you might say:

"I know you are angry."
"I am sorry you are disappointed."

EXAMPLES OF POSITIVE SELF-STATEMENTS

Self-Esteem

I am a good person.
I am kind to others.
I am nice looking.
I am deserving of happiness.
I am positive and confident.
I am happy to be me.

I am a hard worker.
I am proud of myself.
I am fun to be with.
I am a nice person.
I am very special.
I am unique.

Reducing Stress

I can meet this challenge.
I can handle this situation.
Made in the shade.
Lighten up. Let it go.
Think positively.

I'm in control.
I will be calm and relaxed.
Piece of cake.
It will be over shortly.
It wasn't as bad as I expected.

Assertiveness

I will be assertive.
I can speak for myself.
I can make decisions.

I will stand up for myself.
I have certain rights.
I will not be wimpy.

Motivation

I set goals and reach them.
I have a lot of determination.
I can accomplish anything I
    choose.

I have a lot of energy.
I can get things done.
I believe in myself.

Part III

Strategies for Enhancing Self-Respect

Chapter X

IMPROVE ON BODY IMAGE AND PERSONAL ATTRACTIVENESS

How we feel about ourselves is definitely related to how we feel about our bodies. There have been many studies which suggest that one's appearance is an important determiner of self-esteem. It has been found that people who feel negatively about their bodies are also likely to feel negatively about themselves. In other words, if we accept and like our bodies we are more apt to accept and like ourselves. A possible reason for this may be that our ideal self-image includes certain attitudes about our ideal body image. We all have a fairly clear idea of how we would like to look. If we come close to conforming to this ideal body image, we tend to view ourselves in more positive ways. If we deviate too far from our ideal body image, our self-esteem suffers.

In 1985, *Psychology Today* surveyed 30,000 people about their body image. They found that 34% of the men and 38% of the women did not like their looks. The dissatisfaction mainly involved weight. Forty-one percent of the men wanted to weigh less, and 55% of the women felt they were overweight. If the studies are correct about the connection between self-esteem and body image, many Americans have poor self-concepts. However, there are many factors which determine a person's level of self-esteem. A well-rounded individual also derives esteem from integrity, satisfying relationships, creativity, and feelings of accomplishment. But body image does play an important role, partly because it has an effect on the nature of responses a person receives from others.

For persons with developmental disabilities an attractive body image can positively influence social acceptance and self-respect. It can also lead to more favorable work relationships and increased opportunities for interaction with the nondisabled. Unfortunately, it is a reality that there is prejudice against those who look "strange" or "different." Studies indicate that in interactions between the nondisabled and persons with disabilities, the nondisabled people were physically nervous and inhibited and they would terminate interactions sooner than they would have with another nondisabled individual. For those with physical handicaps the signs of disablement are obvious: wheelchairs, walkers, crutches, and the like. For persons with developmental disabilities there are certain physical cues which are not as obvious, yet are discernable. These cues may include clothes, hairstyles, or makeup that is not age appropriate or well chosen, or facial hair or adaptive equipment which is out of the ordinary. These problems, as well as some types of facial disfigurement, can be changed or improved upon. Before elaborating on these ideas, it is important to first discuss two other issues which greatly influence self-respect and body image. They are inner beauty and self-acceptance.

Inner Beauty

Inner beauty is an emotional wealth that transcends physical attractiveness. A person's inner beauty is evident in the special way he relates to others. He is warm and kind and always willing to listen or lend a hand. The authors know a lovely woman named Louise who has this special quality. There is a certain calmness and gentleness about Louise. People always feel comfortable and at ease around her. She is compassionate and giving and is always thinking of the comfort and welfare of others. And although sensitive and, at times, vulnerable, you can feel a special strength and courage within her. Louise's inner beauty touches everyone around her. It is what makes her such a unique person.

Self-Acceptance

Healthy, positive self-respect and self-esteem must also include self-acceptance. We all have strengths, weaknesses, and limitations. If we focus only on our weaknesses, our self-esteem will most certainly suffer. If we focus only on our strengths and deny or disown our limitations, then our self-appraisal will be distorted. We must strive to integrate both our strengths and weaknesses into a total picture of ourselves. With such awareness we can be self-accepting. This does not mean we cannot work to improve our weaknesses. But expectations for improvement must be based on realistic possibilities. In working with persons with developmental disabilities to gain self-acceptance, the following guidelines may be helpful:

1. Call attention to their strengths and abilities. Help them to talk openly about what they like and value about themselves. Take a photograph or have

them draw a picture of a situation where they are demonstrating a skill or doing something well. Suggest that they put the picture up in their room to remind them of their abilities.

2.   Assist them in identifying their weaknesses.
     Gently work to bring their frustrations to the surface. If possible, set goals to improve on these weaknesses or limitations. Explain to them that everyone has shortcomings. Give examples of the weaknesses of people they admire. Tell them that in life we all must learn to live with our limitations.

3.   Help them to share emotionally in the gifts of others, without regretting their own limitations.
     Encourage them to take pride in knowing (or being a fan of) someone who has a special ability. Take them to the athletic event or other activity where that person may be performing. Teach them to be a supporter and encourager of others, as well as themselves.

Improving Body Image

Enhancing body image and feelings of personal attractiveness in individuals can have a dramatic effect on self-esteem and self-respect. Teachers and professionals should use any special knowledge they have, as well as the following guidelines:

1. Discuss with the person his feelings about his body (i.e., strengths, weaknesses).
    Help him to talk about his insecurities and frustrations. Ask him how he would ideally like to look in terms of weight, skin, or hairstyle. Also, discuss what he likes in regard to clothes and current styles. Set goals based on his preferences as well as your suggestions.

2. Assist them in valuing their own uniqueness. Persons with disabilities (like everyone) are constantly inundated by conventional notions of beauty in magazines and on television commercials. They may develop feelings of inferiority if they compare themselves to these "Madison Avenue" images. Emphasize to them that they should avoid

making comparisons with others because everyone is beautiful and attractive in their own unique way.

3. Help them to enhance their physical attractiveness.
A. Clothing
Clothes make an important statement about a person's attitude and self-image. Whenever possible, clothes should be flattering and not simply "functional." Colors and styles should be in harmony with a person's coloring and body type. Always accent strengths and downplay weaknesses. For example, a woman in a wheelchair who has experienced muscle atrophy in her legs would look better in a long, full skirt as opposed to the current style of short, tight skirts. For practicality, velcro snaps can aid a person in self-dressing. Also, strengthened seams, heavier material, and elbow and knee patches can help to preserve garments that receive a great deal of wear.

B. Make-up and hairstyles
All young women desire to maximize their positive features. Young women with developmental disabilities are no different. The appropriate application of make-up (color, amount, and

placement) can enhance eyes, lips and facial features. These techniques are not easy to learn, and it can be helpful for parents and professionals to seek professional cosmetic evaluations and training for the person. Additionally, a cute hairstyle can be a positive. Unfortunately, it is not always best to follow current styles. A young woman with cerebral palsy may not be capable of managing a current hair fashion. It will be important to find an easy-to-care-for style and for her to accessorize with current jewelry and dress to bring her into current style. It can be more stigmatizing to try to carry out a fashion-fad statement and fail than to have a simple hairstyle, conservatively managed, allowing the person to be presented appropriately groomed.

C. Plastic surgery

While plastic surgery has long been a medical technique used to improve physical anomalies such as cleft lip and palate and other cranial facial deformities, it has recently become a procedure used with persons with Down syndrome.

Facial plastic surgery in persons with Down syndrome
has included tongue reduction, lower lip reduction,
chin implants, nasal implants, epicanthal z-plasty,
lateral canthoplasty, removal of fat tissue from the
anterior neck area, and otoplasty. (Hohler, 1977;
Lanigan, 1985). Prosthetic dental procedures have
also been used. (Talches, Sela, Lewin-Epstein,
Wexler, and Peled, 1984).

There are two goals in facial plastic surgery: to make
the person's physical appearance more normal and to
improve the person's general functioning. In the case
of Down syndrome, it is well accepted that plastic
surgery can indeed produce changes in the facial
appearance. Photographic evidence by Olbrisch
(1982), Wexler and Peled (1983), and Lemperle
(1985) supports the statement that marked changes are
possible.

Changes in functioning are more difficult to support.
Children may have problems related to tongue
movements (as is known to some persons with Down
syndrome), feeding problems and speech difficulties.
While some parents have reported improvements in

these areas as well, further controlled studies are still needed to measure the effects of such surgical techniques.

Another challenge has been offered by one of the medical leaders in the field of Down syndrome. Pueschel (1984) argued that such surgery is required only if the child has a significant deformity. He challenged the view that the physical characteristics of Down syndrome are deformities. A survey by Pueschel of parents' and physicians' perceptions in regard to facial features resulted in physicians being more likely to regard the features of Down syndrome negatively.

While much controversy still remains around this issue, the authors of the book feel plastic surgery is an option to be considered in cases of abnormal deformities but would exclude Down syndrome as a deformity.

D. Proper diet and exercise.
Eating nutritious foods and staying away from fat, sugar and salt is good advice for anyone. If a person

uses a wheelchair, it may be easy for him to put on weight around the middle. He must be especially careful of high calorie foods. Exercise in the form of swimming or specialized aerobics is very good for the cardiovascular system and also is extremely effective in burning off unwanted pounds. Regular exercise must be taught. It is as important as a living or vocational skill program. The results have life enhancing qualities.

Chapter XI

ESTABLISH MEANINGFUL FRIENDSHIPS

Friendships fulfill a deep need we all have in our lives to be loved and accepted. A good friend will allow us to be ourselves. We can share with him what we think, feel, and value and what we believe in and are committed to. The very act of sharing these feelings with another person leads to a meaningful friendship. Common interests, shared goals and hobbies, and mutual respect also help the relationship to flourish. We naturally feel better about ourselves when we have others in our lives who love and accept us. Good friends and the sense of connectiveness they provide is essential to healthy self-respect and self-esteem.

A good friend can be hard to find for persons with a developmental disability. They may be isolated and overprotected and have very few opportunities to form friendships. Even when they are in a position to meet new people, they may be painfully shy and unassertive or overly anxious and awkward. Many individuals with developmental disabilities simply lack "friendship skills." Without the experience of having friends, it is difficult to know how to relate to friends. Friendship skills include sharing, being a good listener, being respectful and caring, and showing a willingness to compromise and apologize when we are wrong. When teachers and professionals help to teach such skills, they are passing on an invaluable gift.

There are three key ingredients to a successful and enduring relationship. The first is the capacity to share places. By places we mean a similar school, vocational program site, swimming pool, recreation center, any place where the two friends share a common environment. This promotes shared experiences because the friends may know some of the same people and do similar things. The second ingredient is sharing interests or hobbies, and may come as a result of sharing places. Shared interests may include music, sports, movies, art or hobbies such as gardening, collecting things or building model airplanes. Having a similar interest or hobby often leads to doing the activity together and strengthening a friendship.

The third ingredient of a good friendship involves perceiving a competency in the other person. For example, in a friendship between a nondisabled person and a person with a disability, each party must see a strength or ability in the other. If the nondisabled person does not see a competency in the person with a disability, the friendship may simply be a "helper" relationship. This is one of the reasons why it is so important for the parent, teacher, or professional to help the child or adolescent with a developmental disability to develop a unique or unusual skill. Such a skill might involve becoming an expert at computer games, ping pong, or even being especially good at maneuvering a power wheelchair. Any competence that displays a uniqueness or special ability will help to create a successful friendship.

The decision to form a friendship with someone is greatly influenced by a first impression. In the first thirty seconds that we meet a new person we make a judgment. Either we like them and want to see them again or we feel nothing in particular and are indifferent about pursuing a friendship. Having a disability can actually work to one's advantage. Because individuals with disabilities stand out in a crowd, people remember them. This means they may have a chance of making a positive first impression that won't be easily forgotten. The process of making a good impression is dependent on the kinds of positive messages we send out. People with developmental disabilities would benefit from the following guidelines in the art of meeting and greeting others:

1. Smile.

    A smile costs nothing but means everything. It gives people the impression that you're open, friendly, and approachable. A smile also lets others know that you're a happy, positive individual, the kind of person other people would want to get to know.

2. Maintain eye contact.

    People who can't look other people in the eye appear to be hiding something. They also seem passive and unattentive. People who do have good eye contact make others feel they're being listened to and understood.

3. Ask people about themselves.

    Pretend you're a TV interviewer like Oprah Winfrey or Phil Donahue. Ask people about their jobs, or how they like where they live, or what kind of hobbies or

interests they have. You'll find that people love to
talk about themselves.

4. Be a good listener.
    People need to feel they're being listened to. It makes
    them feel that their ideas and opinions really matter.
    And it shows them that they are valued and respected
    as people. Repeat back things they have said, in your
    own words, so they'll know you're listening.

5. Compliment people in a sincere way.
    No one ever hears enough nice things about
    themselves. Let a person know if you like something
    about them. It is not just flattery when you really
    mean it. Just think how nice you feel when you hear a
    sincere compliment from someone.

In his book *How to Have a Friend and Be a Friend*,
Bry (1979) compiled the following list in response to the
question, "What are desirable qualities in a friend?"

*   Someone who will always be there when you need
    him (you can count on, depend on).

- Someone who will do something for you without asking for anything in return.
- Someone you really trust, who takes responsibility for telling you the truth.
- Someone to share your happiness and sadness, your good times and bad times.
- Someone who listens and hears what you're saying.
- Someone who is easy to be with; who cares about you and accepts you as you are.

Teachers and professionals could use this list to promote and direct a discussion of how a good friend acts and behaves. They could ask questions like, "What does it mean to really trust someone?" or "How can we be good listeners?" A question could also be asked about "best friends" or "special friends:" How did she become your best friend and what is it that makes her special?

The second author of this book has had nearly a life-long friendship with a man named David who has Down syndrome. This friendship began because they shared places: a neighborhood, the park, the area's public swimming pool. Over the years, special hobbies and interests have bonded them: a love for classical music, bike riding, playing cards and gardening.

Their friendship is beautiful and it is David's ability to be a friend that has nourished the friendship.

his listening heart
his honest expression of feelings
and appreciations
his gift of self
his spontaneous smiles
and his faithfulness
That's what makes him a special friend!

Chapter XII

CLARIFY VALUES

In building a new home, one of the first considerations is to decide on a house plan. After studying the house plan and making any desired adjustment, it is then converted into a blueprint. The blueprint reflects choices we have made regarding the size of the house, the number of bedrooms, the placement of the doors and windows, and many other decisions. It guides the builders in the construction of the new home. Values serve a similar purpose in the way they guide our lives. They reflect choices we make regarding our friends, family, career and lifestyle. Values represent our system of personal ethics, telling us what is "right" and "wrong" in life. If we operate in accordance with our values and personal ethics, our self-worth stays high and so does our self-respect. If we behave in confict with our stated values then we lose the respect of others, as well as ourselves.

A well-defined value system is also important for persons with developmental disabilities. It provides them with a valuable blueprint or framework for making decisions in relationships, at work, in the community and in their home environment. A strong sense of values also serves as a guide for moral decision-making. It can be an important tool for avoiding sexual exploitation and in making choices regarding birth control, marriage, and parenthood. For the most part, it has been assumed that persons with developmental disabilities don't have the ability to make moral decisions because of diminished cognitive functioning. This has been proven false by a number of studies (Mahoney and Stephens, 1974; McLaughlin and Stephens, 1974; Moore and Stephens, 1974; Stephens and McLaughlin, 1974) which indicate that people with developmental disabilities do improve over time on tests of moral judgment and conduct.

For teachers and professionals the challenge is to create methods of teaching values clarification whch are both practical and informative. One such method was designed specifically for persons with developmental disabilities by an educator named Dr. Alexander Tymchuk. It is a board game called "Consequences" (Ednick Communications) and helps those with developmental disabilities to develop values and learn about the options they have in making decisions. In one stage of the game called "Super Consequences," players spin in order to pick from stacks of cards. The cards are categorized according to community, work, and home, and involve certain social skills or situations. If the brief description on the card indicates positive or appropriate behavior, the player advances a space or two. If the behavior is inappropriate, the player may go backward on the board. For example, from the community category: "A stranger asks your name. You ignore him. Go forward one space." Each card is read aloud to augment the learning process. Since players immediately advance or go backwards on the board, they are able to learn which behaviors are "right" and which are "wrong." And, because it is done in a game format, interest and attention are maintained. The following are other sample items from the "Consequences" game:

Community category

- Some friends try to get you to take a pill. You don't. Go forward 2 spaces and collect a bonus card.
- You go on a jog-a-thon to aid the blind. Go forward 1 space and collect a bonus card.
- You push your way to the front of the line at a movie. Go back 1 space.

- You found a wallet and mailed it to the owner. Go forward 2 spaces and collect a bonus card.

Work category

- You admit leaving early. Stay where you are.
- Your friend brings beer to work. You refuse to have any. Go forward 2 spaces and collect a bonus card.
- When you come to the lunch room everyone becomes quiet. You do not think they are talking about you. Go forward 1 space.
- You do not apologize for being late and your boss gets mad. Go back 1 space.

Home category

- Your roommate called you stupid. You ignore her. Go forward 1 space.
- You picked up litter in front of your apartment, and the manager thanks you. Go forward 2 spaces.
- Your roommate forgot his wallet. You pay for lunch. Go forward 1 space.
- You slam the door in anger. Miss 1 turn.

Dr. Tymchuk's "Consequences" game helps the person with a developmental disability to clarify values through learning how to respond appropriately in certain interpersonal situations. Other values clarification exercises are not as focused on content but instead emphasize creating a process whereby individuals can learn to make choices and decisions. Persons with developmental disabilities can benefit from both approaches. Teachers and professionals should use tangible, practical examples as well as guidelines for decision-making. They should also directly discuss values with the person and reinforce him for making responsible choices.

At the fiber of many persons' values are the moral and ethical teachings of their church. Young people with developmental disabilities have often been overlooked in the church with few special programs designed to teach them God's love and God's plan for all our lives.

We live in a time when the old laws of morality can seem irrelevant, and the new ethics and values seem ambiguous. The home, church and community are going to have to form a partnership if we are to help persons with developmental disabilities approach moral decision making.

When we feel loved by God we feel good about ourselves and can feel we are His special unique creation. When we have self-confidence and self-respect, we can live moral, inner-directed lives in line with Judeo-Christian beliefs.

Persons with developmental disabilities can learn to live exemplary lives. They will learn best by example. If we want them to know the great power of self-acceptance then we will have to practice personally and professionally God's indispensable acceptance and love.

If we model our beliefs, we will serve as examples in our churches, our community and our own homes and in so doing, release more of God's love in the world—that's self-esteem in action.

Appendices

Appendix I
SELF-ESTEEM ASSESSMENT

		Always	Most of the Time	Some of the Time	Never
1.	I like to try new things.	4	3	2	1
2.	I let people know how I feel.	4	3	2	1
3.	I set goals.	4	3	2	1
4.	I try to be independent.	4	3	2	1
5.	I can handle stress.	4	3	2	1
6.	I get things done.	4	3	2	1
7.	I like the way I look.	4	3	2	1
8.	I am proud of my accomplishments.	4	3	2	1
9.	I am an honest person.	4	3	2	1
10.	I have good friends.	4	3	2	1
11.	I get along OK with my parents.	4	3	2	1
12.	I am a good person.	4	3	2	1

Scoring: The total numerical score on this test is not important. The items are to be assessed individually in order to pinpoint strengths and weaknesses. The first 6 items pertain to issues of self-confidence while the final 6 items involve questions of self-respect. It is an informal evaluation designed to give the teacher or professional a basic idea of what general areas of self-esteem could be improved upon.

Appendix II

REFERENCES

Branden, N. (1969). *The Psychology of Self-Esteem*, pp. 110-113. New York: Bantam Books, Inc.

Bry, A. (1979). *How to Have a Friend and Be a Friend*. New York: Bry, Inc.

Canfield, J. and Wells, H.C. (1976). *100 Ways to Enhance Self-Esteem in the Classroom: A Handbook for Parents and Teachers*. New Jersey: Prentice-Hall, Inc.

Helmstettler, Shad. (1986). *What to Say When You Talk to Yourself*. Scottsdale, Arizona: Grindle Press.

Hohler & Lanigan (1985). Reconstructive facial surgery. *Australian and Zealand Journal of Developmental Disabilities*. Vol. 8, No. 1.

Mahoney, E.J., Jr. and Stephens, B. (1974). Two year gains in moral judgment by normals and retardates. *American Journal of Mental Deficiency, 79*, 131-141.

Maslow, A. H. (1954). *Motivation and Personality*, p. 45. New York: Harper and Row Publishers, Inc.

McLaughlin, J.A. and Stephens, B. (1974). Interrelationships among reasoning, moral judgment, and moral conduct. *American Journal of Mental Deficiency, 79,* 147-153.

Moore, G. and Stephens, B. (1974). Two year gains in moral conduct by normals and retardates. *American Journal of Mental Deficiency, 79,* 147-153.

Pueschel, S.M. (1984). *The Young Child with Down Syndrome.* New York: Human Sciences Press.

Stephens, B. and McLaughlin, J.A. (1974). Two year gains in moral conduct by normals and retardates. *American Journal of Mental Deficiency, 79,* 116-126.

Talches, Sala and Lewin-Epstein (1986). Facial surgery. *Australian and Zealand Journal of Developmental Disabilities.* Vol. 8. No. 2.

Wexler, M.R.; Mintzker, Y. and Peled, I.J. (1984). Reconstructive facial surgery in Down syndrome. *Journal of the Israel Medical Association.* Vol, XCIII. No. 3-4.